The Untold Story of

DISEASE X

The Invisible Foe - What You Need to Know to Protect Yourself and Others

Dr. Nelk

Table of contents

Introduction

In the vast landscape of infectious diseases that humanity grapples with, there exists an enigmatic entity known as Disease X. It's not a tangible foe with a face, but rather a cryptic term coined by the World Health Organization (WHO) to represent a hypothetical, unknown pathogen that could unleash a future epidemic.

Disease X made its debut in 2018 when the WHO, in its pursuit of bolstering global preparedness, added this mysterious entity to its shortlist of blueprint priority diseases. But what exactly is Disease X, and why does it warrant our attention?

Imagine Disease X as a shadowy figure lurking in the background, representing the potential for a serious international epidemic caused by a pathogen currently unknown to cause human disease. Its inclusion in the list was not an arbitrary decision but a calculated move to encourage flexibility in planning and preparedness. The goal was clear: to ensure that our defense mechanisms, including vaccines and diagnostic tools, are adaptable enough to respond swiftly to the unforeseen.

As we embark on this journey to unravel the story of Disease X, we delve into the genesis of this term, understanding why it was named, and exploring the rationale behind its existence. Through this exploration, we aim to shed light on the urgency of comprehending the unknown, preparing ourselves for an invisible adversary that may shape the future of global health. The tale of Disease X is not just a narrative of potential threats; it is a call to action, beckoning us to navigate the uncharted territories of infectious diseases and fortify our defenses against the unseen.

Significance and urgency of understanding and preparing for the unknown pathogen

In the grand tapestry of global health, the significance of understanding and preparing for the unknown pathogen, embodied by Disease X, cannot be overstated. It's a call to vigilance, an urgent plea to recognize the gravity of the unseen peril that looms on the horizon.

The world witnessed the devastating consequences of unpreparedness during the Ebola epidemic of 2014-2016, where over 11,000 lives were lost due to the lack of rapid and effective medical countermeasures. This crisis served as a wake-up call, prompting the World Health Organization (WHO) to take proactive measures and introduce the concept of Disease X to its priority list in 2018.

Disease X is not merely a hypothetical construct; it's a manifestation of the unpredictable nature of infectious diseases. The term encapsulates the potential for an unknown pathogen to incite an international epidemic, catching us off guard and challenging our existing medical arsenal. As we grapple with the aftermath of the COVID-19 pandemic, the urgency to prepare for the next unknown threat becomes even more apparent.

Flexibility in planning is paramount. The rigidity of focusing solely on known pathogens leaves us vulnerable to the ever-evolving landscape of infectious diseases. Disease X compels us to broaden our perspective, encouraging the development of versatile platforms for vaccines, drug therapies, and diagnostic tests. It's a strategic move to ensure that our response mechanisms are not confined to specific strains but are nimble enough to adapt to unforeseen adversaries.

To prepare for Disease X is to acknowledge the unpredictable nature of infectious diseases. It's an investment in our collective resilience, a commitment to fortify our defenses against an invisible foe. As we navigate the intricacies of this unknown pathogen, the significance lies not just in deciphering its potential threats but in fostering a global mindset of preparedness, collaboration, and a steadfast determination to face the unseen with unwavering resilience.

Chapter 1:

The Genesis of Disease X

In the intricate realm of global health, the World Health Organization's (WHO) Research and Development (R&D) Blueprint serves as a compass, guiding efforts to anticipate and counteract emerging infectious diseases. The genesis of Disease X lies intertwined with the inception of this strategic blueprint.

In the wake of the 2014-2016 Ebola epidemic in West Africa, a stark realization echoed through the global health community—the urgent need for a proactive and comprehensive approach to tackle potential pandemics. The WHO responded by establishing the R&D Blueprint, a visionary initiative aimed at accelerating the development of medical countermeasures for high-priority diseases.

The R&D Blueprint was not crafted in isolation; instead, it involved a collaborative effort with member organizations and a pool of global experts. This collective endeavor birthed a shortlist of less than ten blueprint priority diseases, featuring well-known adversaries like Ebola, Zika, and SARS. However, recognizing the unpredictable nature of infectious diseases, the WHO took a bold step in 2018 by adding Disease X to this exclusive list.

The creation of Disease X within the R&D Blueprint was not a proclamation of a specific threat but a recognition of the potential for an unknown pathogen to plunge the world into an international epidemic. It was a strategic move to challenge the scientific community to prepare for an unseen adversary, urging them to develop flexible and adaptable tools that could respond rapidly to unforeseen strains.

As Disease X took its place on the blueprint, the WHO sent a resounding message—that our preparedness should not be confined to known pathogens alone. Instead, it should encompass a broader spectrum, a vigilant stance against the unknown. The R&D Blueprint, with Disease X at its core, stands as a testament to the WHO's commitment to fostering resilience and innovation in the face of emerging infectious threats. The story of Disease X is not just a narrative of anticipation; it is an evolving chapter in the ongoing saga of global health, where adaptability and preparedness reign supreme in the quest to outsmart the unseen.

Evolution of the shortlist of blueprint priority diseases

The evolution of the shortlist of blueprint priority diseases within the World Health Organization's (WHO) Research and Development (R&D) Blueprint is akin to a dynamic dance—a responsive and ever-changing choreography shaped by the ebb and flow of emerging infectious threats.

The journey began in May 2015 when, in the midst of pandemic preparations preceding the COVID-19 era, the WHO was tasked with crafting an R&D Blueprint for Action to

Prevent Epidemics. The goal was clear: to bridge the gap between the identification of viral outbreaks and the approval of vaccines and treatments, thereby thwarting the escalation of these outbreaks into public health emergencies.

A cohort of global experts, known as the R&D Blueprint Scientific Advisory Group, assembled to draft a shortlist of less than ten blueprint priority diseases. This list was not static; rather, it underwent an annual metamorphosis, a reflection of the ever-evolving landscape of infectious diseases.

Since 2015, the shortlist has been a canvas painted with the hues of both well-known adversaries and geographically specific challenges. Diseases like Ebola, Zika, and SARS found their place alongside more localized threats such as Lassa fever, Marburg virus, Rift Valley fever, and Nipah virus.

The rationale behind this curated selection was to focus on the most serious emerging infectious diseases for which preventive options were scarce. Each annual update was a meticulous curation, balancing the recognition of known threats with the anticipation of the unknown.

In February 2018, a pivotal moment occurred—the inclusion of Disease X to this exclusive list. The shortlist, now enriched with the enigmatic Disease X, became a testament to the WHO's foresight. It acknowledged the potential for a future epidemic caused by an unknown pathogen, challenging the global health community to fortify its preparedness against the unseen.

As we trace the evolution of the shortlist, it is not merely a chronicle of diseases; it is a narrative of adaptability, foresight, and the relentless pursuit of resilience in the face of ever-changing microbial landscapes. The shortlist, with Disease X at its heart, embodies the WHO's commitment to a proactive and dynamic approach in the ongoing battle against emerging infectious threats.

Chapter 2:
Disease X Unveiled

In the intricate tapestry of infectious diseases, there exists a phantom—a mysterious entity with the potential to alter the course of human history. It is not a defined nemesis but a concept, a placeholder in the lexicon of global health—the enigmatic Disease X.

Imagine Disease X not as a specific foe but as a manifestation of the unpredictable nature of infectious threats. Coined by the World Health Organization (WHO) in February 2018, Disease X represents a hypothetical, unknown pathogen that could be the harbinger of a future epidemic. It's a term designed not to instill fear but to instigate preparedness—a call to arms in the face of an unseen adversary.

The genesis of Disease X lies in the aftermath of the 2014-2016 Ebola epidemic, a period that laid bare the vulnerabilities in our global health defense mechanisms. The WHO, recognizing the need for a proactive strategy, introduced the Research and Development (R&D) Blueprint—an initiative aimed at expediting the creation of medical countermeasures for high-priority diseases.

Disease X was not added to the blueprint as a concrete entity but as a symbolic acknowledgment of the potential for an unknown pathogen to cause an international epidemic. It challenged scientists and researchers to think beyond the known adversaries like Ebola, Zika, and SARS, urging them to develop flexible platforms for vaccines, therapies, and diagnostics.

This hypothetical pathogen, residing in the realm of the unknown, serves as a reminder that our preparedness should not hinge solely on what we know but extend to what we might encounter. Disease X is a narrative of anticipation, a storyline that unfolds in the gaps between familiar threats, pushing the boundaries of scientific preparedness.

The role of Disease X in encouraging flexible planning and broad countermeasures

In the intricate dance between science and the unseen, Disease X emerges as a silent orchestrator, compelling the global health community to reevaluate its strategies and embrace flexibility in the face of uncertainty.

Coined by the World Health Organization (WHO) in February 2018, Disease X is not just a hypothetical pathogen; it is a catalyst for change, a symbolic reminder that our preparedness should transcend the boundaries of the known and extend into the uncharted realms of potential threats. At its core, Disease X plays a pivotal role in encouraging flexible planning and the development of broad countermeasures.

The traditional approach to infectious diseases often involves tailoring responses to specific known threats—identifying a pathogen, studying its characteristics, and developing targeted countermeasures.

However, Disease X challenges this paradigm. It nudges scientists and researchers to think beyond the familiar, to anticipate the unexpected, and to craft strategies that can adapt to the ever-changing landscape of infectious threats.

One of the key contributions of Disease X lies in its ability to stimulate the creation of flexible platforms for medical interventions. Instead of focusing solely on individual strains or pathogens, Disease X encourages the development of countermeasures that can be "plug and play," applicable to a wide array of diseases. This approach ensures that when faced with an unknown pathogen, the global health community can respond rapidly with vaccines, drug therapies, and diagnostic tools that are versatile and adaptable.

The role of Disease X extends beyond theoretical planning. It serves as a practical guide, prompting organizations like the WHO to invest in research and development that spans entire classes of viruses. This broader perspective not only enhances our ability to respond to unforeseen strains but also accelerates the pace of scientific innovation.

As we navigate the complexities of infectious diseases, Disease X emerges as a driving force behind a paradigm shift—a shift from reactive responses to proactive, anticipatory strategies. It is a silent protagonist, urging us to embrace adaptability, foster innovation, and be prepared for the unknown. The story of Disease X is not just a tale of a hypothetical pathogen; it is a narrative of resilience, a reminder that in the ever-evolving battle against infectious diseases, flexibility and foresight are our greatest allies.

Chapter 3:

Rationale and Background

Before the world found itself in the relentless grip of the COVID-19 pandemic, there existed a time of pandemic preparations—an era marked by a collective awareness of the potential threats posed by emerging infectious diseases. It was a period when global health organizations, including the World Health Organization (WHO), were tasked with crafting a blueprint for action, a roadmap to navigate the intricate landscape of viral outbreaks.

In May 2015, against the backdrop of the looming specter of infectious diseases, the WHO responded to the call for proactive measures. Member organizations implored the WHO to create a Research and Development (R&D) Blueprint for Action to Prevent Epidemics. The primary objective was clear: to bridge the temporal gap between the identification of viral outbreaks and the approval of vaccines and treatments—a critical endeavor to prevent these outbreaks from escalating into public health emergencies.

This blueprint was not a static document but a dynamic initiative that evolved annually. The WHO assembled a group of global experts, the R&D Blueprint Scientific Advisory Group, entrusted with the task of drafting a shortlist of less than ten blueprint priority diseases. These were not just any diseases; they were the most serious emerging infectious diseases for which preventive options were limited.

The annual updates to the shortlist were a reflection of the evolving nature of infectious threats. Diseases like Ebola, Zika, and Severe Acute Respiratory Syndrome (SARS) found a place alongside more geographically specific challenges such as Lassa fever, Marburg virus, Rift Valley fever, and Nipah virus. The goal was to strike a delicate balance between recognizing known adversaries and anticipating the unknown.

It was in this backdrop that the concept of Disease X was introduced in February 2018. As a placeholder for a "knowable unknown" pathogen, Disease X was not a tangible threat but a symbolic acknowledgment of the potential for a future epidemic caused by an unknown pathogen. This addition challenged the global health community to ensure that planning and capabilities were flexible enough to adapt to such an event.

The pandemic preparations before the COVID-19 era laid the groundwork for a paradigm shift—a shift from reactive responses to proactive, anticipatory strategies. It was a time of foresight, a recognition that the battle against infectious diseases required not just knowledge of the known but an acknowledgment of the unknown. Little did the world know that the lessons learned in those preparatory years would become the guiding principles in the face of an unprecedented global health crisis—the era of COVID-19.

The focus on emerging infectious diseases (EIDs) in the R&D Blueprint

In the intricate dance between science and the unseen, the focus on Emerging Infectious Diseases (EIDs) within the Research and Development (R&D) Blueprint for Action became a compass guiding global health efforts. These diseases, often elusive and unpredictable, emerged as central players in the quest for preparedness and rapid response—an acknowledgment that the next viral threat might not be a known adversary but an entity yet to reveal itself.

The genesis of this focus can be traced back to May 2015, a pivotal moment when the World Health Organization (WHO), responding to the urgency of the times, was tasked with crafting a blueprint to prevent epidemics. The emphasis was not on diseases with well-established preventive measures but on those where few options existed—a focus on the most serious EIDs.

A group of global experts, the R&D Blueprint Scientific Advisory Group, took center stage in this endeavor. Their mandate was clear: to draft a shortlist of less than ten blueprint priority diseases. These were not diseases chosen randomly but carefully selected based on the severity of their impact and the lack of effective preventive measures.

Year after year, this shortlist evolved, reflecting the dynamic nature of infectious threats. Diseases like Ebola, Zika, and Severe Acute Respiratory Syndrome (SARS) found a place alongside more region-specific challenges like Lassa fever, Marburg virus, Rift Valley fever, and Nipah virus. The focus on EIDs was not just about recognizing the diseases that had already wreaked havoc; it was about anticipating the potential adversaries yet to emerge.

Within this focus, the R&D Blueprint became a strategic guide, directing attention to the gaps in our preparedness for diseases with the potential to escalate into global emergencies. It was an acknowledgment that the battle against infectious diseases required a proactive stance—an understanding that the landscape of threats was ever-evolving.

As the list of blueprint priority diseases continued to evolve, a subtle but powerful shift occurred. The focus on EIDs was not merely a response to known threats; it was a commitment to preparing for the unknown. This foresight, woven into the fabric of the R&D Blueprint, set the stage for the introduction of Disease X in February 2018—an enigmatic placeholder representing the potential for a serious international epidemic caused by an unknown pathogen.

In the narrative of global health preparedness, the focus on Emerging Infectious Diseases within the R&D Blueprint emerges as a beacon—a guiding principle that urges the world to remain vigilant, adaptive, and ready for the unseen adversaries that may lurk on the horizon. It is a narrative of anticipation, a commitment to stay ahead in the perpetual game of cat and mouse with infectious threats.

Chapter 4:

The WHO's Approach

In the intricate tapestry of global health initiatives, the formation of the Research and Development (R&D) Blueprint Scientific Advisory Group emerged as a critical juncture—a gathering of minds entrusted with the task of navigating the complex terrain of infectious diseases. This group, a confluence of expertise and vision, played a pivotal role in shaping the strategies and priorities that would define the world's preparedness for epidemics.

The genesis of this advisory group can be traced back to May 2015, a time when the World Health Organization (WHO) responded to the pressing need for a proactive approach to epidemics. Member organizations sought the creation of an R&D Blueprint for Action to Prevent Epidemics, a roadmap that would bridge the temporal gap between the identification of viral outbreaks and the approval of vaccines and treatments.

To craft this blueprint, the WHO recognized the necessity of assembling a team of global experts, individuals whose collective knowledge and insights would illuminate the path forward. Thus, the R&D Blueprint Scientific Advisory Group was born—a group with a mandate to draft a shortlist of less than ten blueprint priority diseases. These diseases were not chosen arbitrarily; they were carefully selected based on the severity of their impact and the scarcity of effective preventive measures.

The members of this advisory group became torchbearers in the journey towards preparedness. Their backgrounds spanned diverse fields, from virology to epidemiology, each member bringing a unique perspective to the table. Together, they engaged in a delicate dance of scientific discourse, evaluating the potential threats posed by infectious diseases and identifying gaps in our collective defenses.

Year after year, as the shortlist of blueprint priority diseases evolved, so did the role of the R&D Blueprint Scientific Advisory Group. Their insights became instrumental in shaping not only the list itself but also the broader strategies for addressing emerging infectious diseases. It was a collaborative effort, a synergy of minds committed to staying one step ahead of the ever-changing landscape of infectious threats.

In the narrative of global health preparedness, the formation of this advisory group represents more than just a bureaucratic necessity. It symbolizes a commitment to harnessing the collective wisdom of experts worldwide, recognizing that the battle against infectious diseases requires a multidisciplinary approach. It is a testament to the power of collaboration and the belief that, together, we can fortify our defenses against the unseen adversaries that may test the resilience of humanity.

In the annals of global health strategy, the year 2018 marked a momentous decision—a decision that was not just an addition to a list but a paradigm shift in the way the world approached the looming specter of infectious diseases. It was the year when Disease X, an enigmatic placeholder representing an unknown pathogen with epidemic potential, found its place on the shortlist of blueprint priority diseases within the Research and Development (R&D) Blueprint.

The genesis of this decision can be traced back to the "2018 R&D Blueprint" meeting held in Geneva—a gathering where minds converged to assess the state of global health preparedness and to chart a course for the future. In the wake of this meeting, the World Health Organization (WHO) acknowledged the need to expand the scope of preparedness beyond known adversaries. The concept of Disease X was introduced as a "knowable unknown," a placeholder name signifying the potential for a serious international epidemic caused by an as-yet-unknown pathogen.

The decision to add Disease X to the shortlist was not arbitrary but rooted in a forward-looking approach to global health. It was an acknowledgment that the next big outbreak might be something the world had not encountered before—a realization that history had repeatedly shown the emergence of novel diseases capable of catching the medical world off guard.

At the heart of this decision was the commitment to flexible planning and adaptability. Disease X, as a placeholder, challenged the WHO and the global health community to ensure that their preparedness efforts were not tethered to the familiarity of known pathogens. It urged the development of "plug and play" platforms—technologies and countermeasures that could be swiftly adapted for a wide array of diseases.

The decision was accompanied by a poignant statement from the WHO: "Disease X represents the knowledge that a serious international epidemic could be caused by a pathogen currently unknown to cause human disease." It was a call to action, a recognition that the future of global health would be shaped not only by the diseases we knew but, more crucially, by the ones that remained veiled in uncertainty.

Chapter 5:
Naming Disease X

In the realm of global health, decisions are often imbued with a certain wisdom—a foresight that transcends the immediacy of the present and gazes into the unpredictable terrain of the future. The naming of Disease X, a seemingly cryptic placeholder, was not a mere exercise in nomenclature; it was a strategic move, a manifestation of sagacity aimed at communicating risk and instigating preparedness on a global scale.

The genesis of Disease X as a term can be traced back to the year 2018, a pivotal moment in the evolution of the World Health Organization's (WHO) approach to infectious diseases. As the WHO convened experts and stakeholders to update the shortlist of blueprint priority diseases, a recognition crystallized—a realization that the next major infectious threat might not conform to the familiar names already etched on the list.

In the words of the WHO, Disease X represents the understanding that a serious international epidemic could be sparked by a pathogen currently unknown to cause human disease. The nomenclature, with its enigmatic 'X,' serves as a metaphor for the unknown—an acknowledgment that the identity of the next global health adversary remains elusive, shrouded in the complexities of the microbial world.

This act of naming Disease X, as described by Jonathan D. Quick, the author of "End of Epidemics," was a wise communication of risk. It served as a beacon, signaling to the global community that pandemics are not confined to the diseases we are familiar with—they can emerge from the shadows of the unknown. The 'X' became a symbol of anticipation, a placeholder for a potential future threat that demanded attention and preparedness.

While the establishment of the term might, at first glance, seem like a move designed to incite panic, it carries a more profound purpose. Disease X was introduced to get it on people's radars, to shift the narrative from complacency to proactive readiness. It is a reminder that, in the world of infectious diseases, the balance between panic and complacency is delicate, and informed awareness is the key to striking that balance.

In the grand tapestry of global health, naming Disease X was an act of wisdom that transcended semantics. It was a rallying cry for preparedness, a call to navigate the uncertainties of the microbial world with a resilience fortified by knowledge and foresight. The 'X,' once a symbol of the unknown, became a symbol of readiness—an acknowledgment that our best defense against the unseen lies in our ability to plan and adapt, even in the face of uncertainty.

In the delicate dance of managing global health crises, communication plays a pivotal role. The goal is not just to disseminate information but to strike a delicate balance—a balance between communicating the gravity of a potential threat and averting the twin pitfalls of panic and complacency. In the case of Disease X, this delicate equilibrium became the lodestar guiding the communication strategy.

The introduction of Disease X as a term was not a proclamation of imminent doom; rather, it was a calculated move to communicate risk. The 'X' symbolized the unknown, a placeholder for a pathogen that could potentially trigger a serious international epidemic. However, the messaging around Disease X was crafted with a dual purpose—to raise awareness without inducing unwarranted panic and to foster a sense of urgency without breeding complacency.

Jonathan D. Quick, in his reflections on Disease X, emphasized the wisdom in communicating risk. It was not about sowing fear but about ensuring that the global community was cognizant of the unpredictable nature of infectious diseases. Disease X became a narrative tool, a means to get people's attention and, more importantly, to keep it focused on the need for preparedness.

The 'X,' while enigmatic, was not intended to be a specter of dread. Instead, it served as a symbol of anticipation—a reminder that the next major infectious threat might not adhere to the patterns of the past. The goal was to instill a sense of collective responsibility and readiness, urging nations and communities to be proactive rather than reactive in the face of uncertainty.

In navigating this delicate balance, the narrative around Disease X sought to avoid the extremes. Panic, with its potential for chaos and irrational decision-making, was to be averted. Similarly, complacency, the silent adversary that emerges when familiarity breeds neglect, was to be countered. Disease X, as a communication strategy, aimed to keep the global community in a state of informed alertness—a state where awareness was the antidote to both panic and complacency.

The wisdom behind this approach lies in recognizing that effective communication is not just about conveying information; it is about shaping perceptions and behaviors. Disease X, with its carefully crafted messaging, exemplified a strategic effort to communicate the inherent risks of the microbial world while fostering a collective resolve to confront the unknown with knowledge and preparedness.

Chapter 6:

Disease X Candidates

As we delve into the intricate tapestry of Disease X, it's imperative to explore the potential sources from which this enigmatic threat might emerge. One of the primary suspects in this microbial whodunit is the realm of zoonotic viruses—those elusive pathogens that traverse the boundaries between animals and humans.

Zoonotic viruses, often originating in wildlife, possess the uncanny ability to make the leap from animals to humans, presenting a constant and evolving threat. The World Health Organization (WHO), in its contemplation of Disease X, has identified the zoonotic transmission of viruses as a natural process with significant implications for global health. It's akin to a silent dance between species, where viruses find new hosts, and the intensity of human-animal contact becomes a critical factor.

Professor Marion Koopmans, a WHO special advisor, sheds light on this intricate dance by noting that the rate at which zoonotic diseases appear is accelerating. The modern world, with its increased travel, trade, and encroachment into wildlife habitats, becomes a stage for this dance. The more humans and animals interact, the more opportunities arise for novel viruses to emerge and potentially spark a global health crisis.

On the list of potential candidates for Disease X, the WHO has cited hemorrhagic fevers and non-polio enteroviruses as examples that could emanate from zoonotic sources. The unpredictability lies in the diversity of wildlife reservoirs, each harboring its collection of viruses with the potential to spill over into human populations.

The 'X' in Disease X, therefore, becomes a symbol not just of the unknown pathogen but of the myriad possibilities inherent in the complex interplay between humans and the animal kingdom. It's a recognition that the next global health threat might emerge from the depths of this intricate ecological dance—a dance that demands our vigilance and understanding.

Speculation on specific candidates, such as H7N9 and COVID-19

In the realm of infectious diseases, speculation becomes both a tool for anticipation and a double-edged sword of uncertainty. As we cast our gaze into the speculative horizon of Disease X, certain candidates have emerged, each with its own tale of potential peril.

H7N9 - The Avian Menace:

In the annals of viral threats, the H7N9 "bird flu" virus emerged as a formidable contender. In 2018, this avian influenza strain, with its ominous 38 percent mortality rate, captured the attention of international health authorities. While not officially anointed as Disease X by the World

Health Organization (WHO) or the R&D Blueprint group, the H7N9 virus loomed on the periphery of speculation. Its potential to trigger a global health crisis was likened to the hypothetical nature of Disease X. China's reluctance to share samples of the new H7N9 strain added a layer of intrigue, intensifying concerns that it could be a harbinger of the unknown pathogen that Disease X represents.

COVID-19 - Unmasking the Unknown:
The emergence of COVID-19, caused by the SARS-CoV-2 virus, propelled Disease X from the realm of speculation to a stark reality. In early 2020, as the world grappled with the unprecedented challenges posed by the pandemic, experts and virologists pondered whether COVID-19 could indeed

be the first manifestation of Disease X. Chinese virologist Shi Zhengli, from the Wuhan Institute of Virology, hinted at the connection, suggesting that the first Disease X might be a coronavirus. Marion Koopmans, a member of the WHO's R&D Blueprint Special Advisory Group, echoed these sentiments, describing the outbreak as the first true pandemic challenge fitting the Disease X category. The narrative around COVID-19, therefore, became intertwined with the speculative landscape of Disease X, blurring the lines between the known and the unknown.

In the speculative dance of potential candidates, H7N9 and COVID-19 emerge as protagonists, each with its narrative of threat and uncertainty. The enigma of

Disease X finds echoes in these viral contenders, prompting us to confront the unpredictable nature of infectious diseases and the challenges they pose to global health security. As we navigate this speculative terrain, the shadows of these candidates linger, reminding us that the next chapter in the saga of Disease X may unfold from the seeds of speculation sown in the wake of past pandemics.

Chapter 7:

Disease X in Popular Culture

Beyond the corridors of laboratories and the hushed discussions of scientific symposiums, Disease X finds its way into the realm of public awareness through exhibitions and fictional representations. These avenues serve as both educational tools and imaginative canvases, weaving the narrative of the unknown pathogen into the fabric of our collective consciousness.

Exhibitions:

In 2018, the Museum of London took a bold step by hosting an exhibition titled "Disease X: London's Next Epidemic?" This exhibit, coinciding with the centenary of the Spanish flu epidemic from 1918, sought to bring the specter of an impending epidemic closer to home. Visitors were confronted with the possibility of an unseen adversary, sparking contemplation and raising awareness about the unpredictable nature of infectious diseases. The term "Disease X," once confined to scientific circles, thus made its way into the public arena, challenging individuals to ponder the potential threats lurking in the shadows of global health.

Fictional Representations:

The world of fiction, with its power to captivate and engage, has also embraced the narrative of Disease X. Books such as "Disease" (2020) and "Disease X: The Outbreak" (2019) use the hypothetical concept as a backdrop for exploring the dynamics of global pandemics. These works, while rooted in imagination, serve a dual purpose. They entertain readers with gripping narratives while subtly instilling an awareness of the real-world challenges posed by emerging infectious diseases. The fictionality of these works becomes a conduit for the transmission of knowledge, blurring the lines between speculation and informed awareness.

In the intersection of exhibitions and fiction, Disease X emerges not just as a scientific concept but as a cultural touchpoint. It becomes a subject of contemplation, discussion, and even artistic interpretation. The echoes of these exhibitions and fictional tales resonate, creating a nuanced understanding of the unknown pathogen that lurks in the periphery of our preparedness. As we explore these creative expressions, Disease X transcends its scientific origins, seeping into the collective imagination and urging society to grapple with the potential challenges that may lie ahead.

The impact of Disease X on public perception

The emergence of Disease X, a hypothetical and unknown pathogen, has cast a profound impact on public perception, ushering in a nuanced interplay of curiosity, concern, and a heightened awareness of global health vulnerabilities.

Curiosity as Catalyst:

The mere mention of Disease X acts as a catalyst for curiosity, prompting individuals to delve into the intricacies of a potential pandemic that lies beyond the realm of current knowledge. This curiosity, fueled by a desire for understanding and preparedness, has led to an increased engagement with scientific discourse and a heightened interest in the evolving landscape of infectious diseases. Disease X becomes a focal point of inquiry, inviting individuals to explore the complexities of viral threats and the measures undertaken to counter them.

Concerns and Contemplations:
Simultaneously, Disease X triggers concerns that reverberate through the public sphere. The notion of an unknown pathogen capable of sparking a serious international epidemic introduces an element of uncertainty, challenging conventional perceptions of

health security. Individuals grapple with questions about the unpredictability of future outbreaks and the adequacy of existing preparedness measures. This interplay of concerns becomes a driving force behind discussions on global health governance, research funding, and the need for flexible strategies to combat unforeseen threats.

Heightened Awareness and Preparedness:

Perhaps the most significant impact of Disease X on public perception lies in the heightened awareness of the need for preparedness. The hypothetical nature of this unknown pathogen serves as a call to action, urging communities, governments, and international organizations to fortify their defenses against potential pandemics. The public, now more attuned to the fragility of global health, becomes an active participant in advocating for robust public health infrastructure, rapid response mechanisms, and international collaborations aimed at tackling emerging infectious diseases.

As Disease X permeates public perception, it becomes a prism through which individuals view the intersection of science, public health, and societal resilience. The curiosity it sparks, coupled with the concerns it raises, culminates in a collective awareness that transcends the theoretical boundaries of a hypothetical pathogen. In navigating this landscape of perception, Disease X becomes a narrative thread, weaving through the fabric of public consciousness and leaving an indelible mark on the way we approach the complex tapestry of global health challenges.

Chapter 8:
The Human Element

Amidst the scientific discussions and hypothetical scenarios surrounding Disease X, the narrative gains depth and poignancy when intertwined with personal stories that echo the impact of previous pandemics and outbreaks. These stories, often untold and deeply rooted in the fabric of human experience, serve as poignant reminders of the far-reaching consequences of infectious diseases.

In the aftermath of the 2014–2016 Ebola epidemic in West Africa, the world bore witness to the resilience of communities grappling with the devastating effects of the virus. Personal stories emerged from the heart of the crisis, illustrating the courage of healthcare workers, the strength of families torn apart by illness, and the unwavering spirit of individuals facing an invisible adversary. These narratives not only highlight the challenges faced during a pandemic but also showcase the triumph of the human spirit in the face of adversity.

The echoes of pandemics past reverberate through stories of loss and longing. Families separated by quarantine measures, loved ones lost to the relentless march of infectious diseases—these narratives evoke a profound sense of grief and underscore the human toll exacted by pandemics. Through these personal accounts, the emotional landscape of epidemics becomes palpable, emphasizing the importance of empathy and solidarity in navigating the complexities of global health crises.

Amidst the chaos of pandemics, the stories of frontline heroes emerge as beacons of inspiration. Healthcare workers, often thrust into the epicenter of outbreaks, share their experiences of tireless dedication, selflessness, and the relentless pursuit of saving lives. These personal narratives shed light on the sacrifices made by those on the front lines, portraying a vivid picture of the human side of epidemic response.

In the face of adversity, communities come together, and acts of kindness shine through the darkness. Stories of neighbors supporting one another, strangers extending a helping hand, and collective efforts to mitigate the impact of outbreaks showcase the resilience inherent in human connections. These tales of compassion and solidarity offer a counterpoint to the challenges posed by pandemics, illustrating the strength that emerges when communities unite.

As we navigate the complex landscape of Disease X, these personal stories serve as poignant reminders that behind the statistics and scientific discussions are real lives, real emotions, and real resilience.

The emotional connection to Disease X and its implications

The emotional connection to Disease X transcends the realm of theoretical pandemics, weaving a tapestry of fear, hope, and introspection that resonates deeply with individuals worldwide. As the hypothetical pathogen takes center stage in global health discourse, its emotional implications evoke a spectrum of sentiments that mirror the complexity of the human experience.

At the heart of the emotional connection to Disease X lies an undercurrent of fear and uncertainty. The prospect of an unknown pathogen capable of triggering a serious international epidemic instills a sense of trepidation, challenging the innate human desire for predictability and control. This fear, rooted in the unknown, becomes a powerful force shaping perceptions, behaviors, and the collective psyche.

Conversely, the emotional response to Disease X is not devoid of hope. The hypothetical nature of this unseen foe becomes a catalyst for proactive measures and preparedness. Individuals and communities, spurred by the prospect of a future pandemic, find hope in the collective efforts to strengthen healthcare systems, advance medical research, and foster global collaborations. The emotional connection becomes a driving force behind endeavors to mitigate potential threats and build a resilient front against unforeseen challenges.

The emotional resonance of Disease X extends to introspection, prompting individuals to reflect on the interconnectedness of our global community. The hypothetical pathogen serves as a mirror, reflecting the vulnerabilities of our shared existence and the imperative for global solidarity. This emotional connection fosters a sense of responsibility towards one another, transcending geographical boundaries and cultural divides.

As discussions around Disease X unfold, empathy becomes a guiding emotional thread. The vulnerability of populations, particularly those with limited access to healthcare resources, elicits empathetic responses. The emotional connection prompts individuals to contemplate the disparities in healthcare infrastructure and advocate for equitable solutions that prioritize the most vulnerable among us.

Emotion also fuels inspiration, particularly in the realm of scientific advancements. The collective emotional response to the potential threat of Disease X propels researchers and innovators to push the boundaries of medical knowledge. The emotional connection becomes a driving force behind breakthroughs in vaccine development, rapid response technologies, and collaborative efforts to tackle emerging infectious diseases.

In navigating the emotional landscape of Disease X, it becomes evident that the hypothetical pathogen is not merely a scientific construct; it is a catalyst for a profound emotional journey. Fear and hope, introspection and empathy, converge to shape a narrative that transcends the theoretical, leaving an indelible mark on the collective consciousness and influencing the way we approach global health challenges.

Chapter 9:
Global Preparations

In the realm of preparedness and anticipation, the global community embarked on a series of simulations and dummy runs to simulate the potential impact of Disease X, a hypothetical pathogen with the potential to unleash a global pandemic. These exercises, conducted by health organizations and experts, sought to unveil insights, identify gaps, and refine strategies in the face of an unforeseen and formidable adversary.

The WHO's Health Emergencies Program:
One notable initiative was spearheaded by the World Health Organization's Health Emergencies Program. In October 2019, an unprecedented "Disease X dummy run" unfolded in New York, bringing together 150

participants from various world health agencies and public health systems. The objective was clear: simulate a global pandemic triggered by Disease X. The scenario unfolded in real-time, allowing participants to immerse themselves in the complexities and challenges that would accompany such an eventuality.

Objectives of the Dummy Run:
The dummy run served multiple purposes. It provided a platform for international collaboration, fostering the exchange of ideas, observations, and best practices in combatting a global pandemic. The simulated scenario allowed participants to stress-test existing response mechanisms, identify potential bottlenecks, and explore innovative solutions. The overarching goal

was to enhance preparedness, ensure swift response mechanisms, and create a blueprint for coordinated global action in the face of a genuine threat.

Realism and Complexity:
What set the Disease X dummy run apart was its commitment to realism and complexity. The scenario was meticulously crafted to mirror the unpredictability and intricacies of a genuine global pandemic. From the rapid spread of the hypothetical pathogen to the socio-economic implications and the strain on healthcare systems, every facet was considered. This commitment to authenticity aimed to provide invaluable insights that could inform real-world strategies when

confronted with an unknown and potentially devastating pathogen.

Observations and Lessons Learned:
As the simulated pandemic unfolded, observations and lessons learned became invaluable takeaways. The interconnectedness of global health systems, the importance of rapid information sharing, and the need for agile decision-making emerged as critical themes. The dummy run underscored the significance of a collaborative and coordinated international response, emphasizing that the challenges posed by Disease X could only be effectively addressed through shared knowledge and resources.

The Psychological Impact:

Beyond the logistical and strategic aspects, the dummy run delved into the psychological impact of a global pandemic. Participants grappled with the emotional toll, ethical dilemmas, and communication challenges that would inevitably accompany such an event. This exploration of the human dimension added depth to the preparedness efforts, acknowledging that addressing a global health crisis involves not only logistical prowess but also a nuanced understanding of human behavior and societal dynamics.

In essence, the Disease X dummy run was more than a mere simulation; it was a collective endeavor to fortify our global defenses against the unknown. As the world grapples with the ongoing challenges of infectious diseases, the insights gleaned from these simulations stand as beacons guiding us towards a future where preparedness, collaboration, and adaptability form the pillars of our response to the unpredictable nature of Disease X.

Ongoing efforts by organizations like CEPI and the creation of research centers

In the relentless pursuit of safeguarding humanity against the elusive threat of Disease X, various organizations have taken decisive actions, ushering in a new era of preparedness and research. Among these trailblazers, the Coalition for Epidemic Preparedness Innovations (CEPI) has emerged as a pivotal force, spearheading efforts to develop innovative solutions and foster global collaboration.

CEPI, a dynamic alliance of public, private, philanthropic, and civil organizations, stands at the forefront of the battle against potential pandemics. With an unwavering commitment to proactively address infectious disease threats, CEPI channels resources and expertise to accelerate the development of vaccines, ensuring that the world is equipped with potent countermeasures to combat emerging pathogens.

One of the cornerstones of CEPI's strategy lies in the promotion of rapid response vaccine platforms. These platforms, supported by a comprehensive $3.5 billion plan, are designed to revolutionize the vaccine development landscape. The goal is ambitious yet essential: to develop new immunizations within a mere 100 days of the emergence of a virus with pandemic potential. This groundbreaking approach seeks to outpace the rapid mutation and spread of potential pathogens, offering a nimble and adaptive defense against the unknown.

The fight against Disease X extends beyond vaccines to encompass a multifaceted approach. Recognizing the importance of advanced research capabilities, the World Health Organization (WHO) has taken a monumental step by establishing the WHO Hub for Pandemic and Epidemic Intelligence in Berlin. This hub serves as a nexus for expediting access to crucial data, developing analytical tools, and constructing predictive models to assess potential threats swiftly.

Nations, too, have risen to the challenge, understanding that a united global front is indispensable. In August 2023, the United Kingdom unveiled plans for a groundbreaking research center located on the Porton Down campus. This facility, dedicated to researching pathogens with the potential to emerge as Disease X, represents a strategic investment in preparedness. Equipped with specialist containment facilities, the center aims to develop tests and potential vaccines within a remarkable 100-day timeframe, should a new threat materialize.

Beyond CEPI and national initiatives, a $5 billion U.S. government initiative named Project NextGen signifies a robust commitment to developing next-generation vaccines and treatments for COVID-19. This forward-looking initiative, coupled with a $262.5 million funding injection for a U.S. national network focused on detecting and responding to public health emergencies, reflects a paradigm shift in our approach to pandemic preparedness.

As these initiatives gain momentum, they weave a tapestry of resilience against the specter of Disease X. The collective endeavors of organizations, nations, and global alliances underscore a shared recognition: the imperative to remain vigilant, collaborative, and innovative in the face of an ever-evolving microbial landscape. In the crucible of these efforts, the seeds of a more prepared and responsive world are sown, cultivating a future where the shadows of unknown pathogens are met with unwavering resolve and cutting-edge solutions.

Chapter 10:
The Road Ahead

Current challenges in preparing for Disease X

Amidst the optimism and concerted efforts to combat Disease X, the journey is not without its challenges. A series of formidable obstacles cast shadows on the path to preparedness, demanding strategic solutions and unwavering commitment from the global community.

One of the critical challenges that looms large is the state of health systems worldwide. Many nations grapple with health infrastructures that are not only depleted but also weakened by the enduring strains of previous pandemics and ongoing healthcare demands. The need for substantial investments in healthcare, bolstering infrastructure, and fortifying healthcare delivery capabilities is glaringly evident.

A rising tide of anti-science sentiments poses a significant hurdle in the journey to Disease X preparedness. Vaccine hesitancy, fueled by misinformation and skepticism, threatens to undermine the effectiveness of crucial immunization campaigns. Addressing this challenge requires a concerted effort to communicate accurate information, engage communities, and build trust in the scientific processes underpinning pandemic preparedness.

As memories of past pandemics fade and immediate risks seem to diminish, there's a risk of governments deprioritizing funding for outbreak detection and preparedness. The cyclic nature of public attention and political focus demands a sustained effort to communicate the ongoing importance of vigilance and investment in preparedness, even in periods of relative calm.

The microbial landscape is dynamic, with pathogens evolving and adapting. Zoonotic threats, originating in wildlife and jumping to humans, present a constant challenge. The intensity of human-animal interactions, coupled with environmental changes, accelerates the risk of new diseases emerging. A proactive approach to understanding and mitigating zoonotic threats is paramount.

Climate change emerges as a compounding factor, altering the migration patterns of animals and influencing the prevalence of vector-borne diseases. The intersection of climate change and disease dynamics adds layers of complexity to the preparedness equation. Adapting strategies to address the health implications of climate change becomes integral to an effective response.

Disparities in healthcare access and resources across different regions amplify the challenges of preparedness. Ensuring equitable access to vaccines, diagnostics, and therapeutic interventions becomes not just a moral imperative but a strategic necessity to prevent the amplification of disease burdens in vulnerable populations.

Navigating these challenges demands a holistic and collaborative approach. From fortifying healthcare infrastructures to combating misinformation, the journey to Disease X preparedness necessitates a resilient and adaptable strategy—one that transcends borders, engages diverse communities, and remains agile in the face of evolving threats. Only through collective action and sustained commitment can the world hope to confront Disease X with the strength and resilience it demands.

The importance of staying updated

In the realm of Disease X preparedness, staying updated is not just a suggestion; it's a lifeline. The landscape of infectious diseases is ever-shifting, marked by the unpredictable emergence of new threats. Thus, maintaining an unwavering commitment to real-time information is paramount for individuals, communities, and policymakers alike.

A crucial aspect of staying ahead of Disease X is the establishment and fortification of real-time surveillance and early warning systems. These systems serve as vigilant guardians, constantly scanning the global health horizon for signals of potential threats. Timely detection allows for swift responses, preventing the escalation of localized outbreaks into full-blown pandemics.

Disease X knows no borders, and neither should the information that guides our response. Global collaboration, facilitated by transparent and open information sharing, becomes the linchpin of an effective defense strategy. Scientific communities, public health agencies, and governments must foster an environment where data flows seamlessly across borders, enabling collective insights that transcend geographical constraints.

In the age of information, storytelling plays a pivotal role in shaping perceptions and influencing decisions. When it comes to Disease X, the narrative should not only be accurate but also ethically crafted. Ethical storytelling involves presenting information truthfully, avoiding sensationalism, and steering clear of fearmongering. The goal is not to instill panic but to empower individuals with knowledge that enables informed decision-making.

Effective communication is a two-way street. Engaging communities in the discourse on Disease X requires more than just disseminating information; it demands empathy and respect. Recognizing diverse perspectives, addressing concerns with sensitivity, and fostering a culture of trust are essential components of a communication strategy that resonates with diverse audiences.

Preparedness is an ongoing journey, and the lessons learned from each outbreak, pandemic, or even the threat of Disease X should be viewed as opportunities for continuous improvement. Cultivating a culture of continuous learning involves not only adapting strategies based on experiences but also actively seeking out new knowledge and insights to refine preparedness approaches.

By embracing these principles—real-time surveillance, global collaboration, ethical storytelling, community engagement, and a commitment to continuous learning—we build a foundation that transcends the uncertainties of Disease X. Staying updated becomes not just a habit but a collective responsibility, a shared commitment to a world where the shadows of unknown pathogens are met with the illuminating power of knowledge and collaboration.

Conclusion

In the intricate dance between humanity and the enigmatic threat known as Disease X, our journey has traversed the realms of preparation, vigilance, and the power of collective knowledge. As we conclude this exploration, let's recap the key points that have woven the fabric of our narrative.

Disease X as a Hypothetical Yet Crucial Concept: Disease X, a term conceived by the World Health Organization (WHO), symbolizes the potential peril lurking in unknown pathogens. It serves as a call to arms for scientists, communities, and policymakers to be prepared for the unforeseen.

The WHO's R&D Blueprint: A Blueprint for Preparedness: The

WHO's Research and Development Blueprint stands as a testament to the commitment to proactive readiness. The shortlist of blueprint priority diseases, with Disease X at its core, reflects a strategic approach to face the ever-evolving landscape of infectious diseases.

Evolution of Preparedness: From Pandemics Past to Disease X: Disease X did not emerge in isolation; it is a product of meticulous pandemic preparations dating back to the time before the COVID-19 era. The focus on emerging infectious diseases and the formation of expert advisory groups paved the way for a comprehensive strategy.

The Wisdom of Naming and Communicating Risk: The decision to name Disease X was a strategic move, fostering awareness without inducing panic. This wisdom in communication acknowledges that a delicate balance must be maintained to engage the public without sowing the seeds of unnecessary fear.

Potential Sources and Candidates: Zoonotic Viruses and Beyond: Disease X's potential sources, including zoonotic viruses, underscore the importance of understanding the intricate relationship between humans and animals. Speculations on candidates like H7N9 and the undeniable impact of COVID-19 emphasize the urgency of preparedness.

Engaging Narratives and Ethical Storytelling:

In the storytelling tapestry of Disease X, narratives have the power to inform, empower, and inspire action. Ethical storytelling, free from sensationalism, ensures that the information shared fosters a culture of responsibility and awareness.

As we stand at the crossroads of possibility and uncertainty, the call to action reverberates. Individuals, communities, and global entities are not mere spectators; they are active participants in the narrative of Disease X.

Your Role in the Tapestry:

- Stay Informed: Embrace the power of knowledge. Stay informed about Disease

X and related developments through reliable sources.

- Promote Collaboration: Recognize that preparedness is a collective endeavor. Encourage collaboration, information sharing, and a united front against potential threats.

- Advocate for Ethical Awareness: Be a torchbearer of ethical storytelling. Advocate for narratives that enlighten without inducing unnecessary fear.

- Embrace Continuous Learning: The journey of preparedness is ongoing. Embrace a mindset of continuous learning, adapting strategies based on experiences and emerging insights.

Disease X is not a prophecy of doom; it is a beacon guiding us toward a future fortified by knowledge, collaboration, and a shared commitment to safeguarding global health. The path forward is illuminated by the collective resolve of individuals and communities to face the unknown with resilience and unity.

In the face of Disease X, we are not passive spectators; we are architects of a resilient future. Together, let us navigate the uncharted waters, armed with the light of awareness and the strength of global solidarity. The journey continues, and our shared commitment will be the compass guiding us through the shadows of uncertainty.

www.ingramcontent.com/pod-product-compliance
Lightning Source LLC
Chambersburg PA
CBHW071208290526
45796CB00008B/185